ECZEMA DIET PLAN GUIDE BOOK

The Eczema Diet: Recipes for Skin Health & Eating Well to Reduce Symptoms of Eczema

REX LEWIS

Table of Contents

INTRODUCTION

Dermatitis, Another Name For Eczema, Is A Common, Long-Lasting Skin Condition That Is Marked By Redness, Itching, Swelling, And Occasionally The Formation Of Tiny, Fluid-Filled Blisters. It Is A Word Used To Describe A Group Of Skin Illnesses That Have Similar Symptoms Rather Than A Single Unique Condition. People Of All Ages Can Get Eczema, And It Can Range In Severity From Moderate To Severe.

• Although The Precise Origin Of Eczema Is Unknown, A Mix Of Immune System, Environmental, And Genetic Variables Are Thought To Play A Role. Individuals Who Have A Family

History Of Allergies, Asthma, Or Eczema May Be More Susceptible To Getting The Illness.

• There Are Various Forms Of Eczema, The Most Prevalent Of Which Is Atopic Dermatitis. Atopic Dermatitis Frequently Starts In Childhood And Is Linked To Hay Fever And Asthma, Among Other Allergic Disorders. Other Forms Include Dyshidrotic Eczema, Which Is Characterized By Tiny Blisters On The Hands And Feet, Nummular Eczema, Which Is Coin-Shaped Areas Of Irritated Skin, And Contact Dermatitis, Which Is Brought On By Skin Contact With Irritants Or Allergens.

• Treatment To Alleviate Symptoms And Preventative Actions Are Usually Combined In The Management Of Eczema. These Can Include Staying Away From Irritants, Taking Care Of Your Skin, Applying Moisturizers, And Taking Oral Or Topical Drugs To Lessen Irritation And Inflammation. Healthcare Professionals May Suggest Systemic Medicines Or Phototherapy In Extreme Situations.

Although It Can Be Difficult To Manage, Eczema Is A Chronic Condition That, With The Right Care And Attention, Can Allow The Majority Of Affected Individuals To Lead Normal, Healthy Lives. People Who Have Eczema Must Collaborate Closely

With Medical Specialists To Create A Customized Management Strategy That Addresses Their Unique Requirements And Triggers.

CHAPTER ONE
What Is Dermatitis?

Dermatitis, Another Name For Eczema, Is A Common Skin Ailment Marked By Redness, Itching, And Inflammation. It Frequently Manifests As A Rash, Though Occasionally Tiny Blisters Filled With Fluid May Also Occur. Eczema Is A Word Used To Describe A Collection Of Illnesses With Comparable Symptoms Rather Than A Single Disorder. Atopic Dermatitis Is The Most Common Type Of Eczema, Although There Are Other Types As Well, Including Contact Dermatitis, Nummular Eczema, And Dyshidrotic Eczema.

• Although The Precise Etiology Of Eczema Is Unknown, Immune System, Environmental, And Genetic Factors Are Thought To Play A Combined Role. People Who Have Allergies, Asthma, Or Eczema In Their Family May Be More Likely To Get The Illness.

• Eczema Symptoms Can Range Greatly In Intensity, From Mild To Severe. Dry Or Sensitive Skin, Red Or Swollen Areas, Severe Itching, And, In Certain Situations, Leaking Or Crusting, Are Typical Symptoms. Although It Can Manifest At Any Age, Childhood Onset Is The Most Prevalent.

• Since Eczema Is A Chronic Disorder, It May Last For A Long Time.

Treatments To Reduce Symptoms And Avoid Problems Are Usually Combined In Management. These Precautions Could Involve Recognizing And Avoiding Triggers, Maintaining Proper Skin Care Practices, Utilizing Moisturizers, And Administering Oral Or Topical Drugs To Lessen Irritation And Inflammation. Medical Practitioners May Suggest Systemic Medicines Or Phototherapy In More Severe Situations.

Even Though Eczema Can Be A Chronic Illness, Many People With It Can Successfully Manage Their Symptoms And Lead Regular Lives With The Right Support And Care. Eczema Sufferers Must Collaborate

Closely With Medical Professionals To Create A Customized Management Strategy That Addresses Their Unique Requirements And Triggers.

Eczema Types

Eczema Comes In A Variety Of Forms, Each Having Unique Traits Of Its Own. The Most Typical Kinds Consist Of:

1. Dermatitis Atopic:

• This Type Of Eczema Is The Most Common And Frequently Starts In Childhood. It Is Linked To A Family History Of Atopic Illnesses Like Hay Fever And Asthma. Atopic Dermatitis Can Affect Many Sections Of The Body And Cause Red, Itchy Rashes In Its Victims.

2. Dermatitis In Contact:

• When The Skin Comes Into Contact With Allergens Or Irritants, Contact Dermatitis Develops. It Can Be Divided Into Two Categories: Allergic Contact Dermatitis, Which Is Brought On By An Allergic Reaction To A Particular Chemical, And Irritant Contact Dermatitis, Which Is Brought On By Exposure To Irritating Substances.

3. Nummular Dermatitis:

• The Hallmark Of This Kind Of Eczema Is Coin-Shaped Areas Of Inflamed Skin. It Can Be Extremely Irritating And Typically Affects The Limbs. Although The Exact Origin Of Nummular Eczema Is Unknown, Dry

Skin, Inflammation, Or Allergies May Be Contributing Factors.

4. Eczema Dyshidrotic:

• **Indications Of Dyshidrotic Eczema:** Hands And Feet That Form Tiny Blisters Filled With Fluid. It May Result In Peeling, Redness, And Irritation. Although The Precise Origin Is Unknown, Stress, Allergies, Or Exposure To Specific Metals May Be Involved.

5. Dermatitis Seborrhea:

• The Scalp, Face, And Upper Chest Are Among The Locations With A High Density Of Oil Glands That Are Typically Affected By Seborrheic Dermatitis. Dandruff And Red, Scaly

Spots Are Commonly Linked To It. Although The Precise Etiology Is Unknown, Variables Including Hormone Fluctuations, Yeast Overgrowth, And Heredity May Be Involved.

6. Dermatitis Stasis:

• Stasis Dermatitis Affects The Lower Legs And Is Associated With Impaired Circulation. People Who Have Venous Insufficiency Or Other Disorders That Cause Blood To Pool In Their Legs Frequently Experience It. Redness, Swelling, And Painful Or Itchy Skin Are Among The Symptoms.

7. Dermatitis Neurodermic:

• Repetitive Scratching Or Rubbing Of The Skin Results In Thickened, Scaly Patches Of Skin Known As Neurodermatitis. It Is Frequently Linked To Psychological Or Stress-Related Issues.

8. The Id Reaction, Or Autoeczematization:

• Autoeczematization, Sometimes Referred To As An ID Reaction, Is An Uncommon Kind Of Eczema That Develops In Reaction To An Infection On The Skin Or Inflammation In Another Area Of The Body. It Causes Extensive Sores That Resemble Eczema.

It's Crucial To Remember That Different People May Have Different Types Of Eczema At The Same Time, And That Each Person's Symptoms And Severity Will Differ. For An Accurate Diagnosis And Suitable Treatment, Speaking With A Healthcare Provider Is Essential For Anyone Who Thinks They May Have Eczema.

Triggers For Eczema

Since Each Person's Eczema Triggers Are Unique, Pinpointing The Right Ones Is Crucial To Controlling And Averting Flare-Ups. Although Each Person's Triggers Are Unique, The Following Common Causes May Contribute To Outbreaks Of Eczema:

1. Allergens:

• Eczema Symptoms Can Be Brought On By Exposure To Allergens Such As Dust Mites, Mildew, Pet Dander, And Pollen. Identifying And Avoiding Contact With Particular Allergens May Aid In The Management Of The Illness.

2. Irritants:

• Some Materials Can Irritate The Skin And Cause Flare-Ups Of Eczema. Typical Irritants Include Specific Materials, Scents, Detergents, And Harsh Soaps. It May Help To Use Gentle, Hypoallergenic Products And Stay Away From Irritants.

3. Dry Skin Type:

• Eczema Is Frequently Triggered By Dry Skin. To Avoid Dryness And Reduce The Chance Of Flare-Ups, It's Essential To Moisturize Your Skin On A Regular Basis.

4. Stress

• Eczema Symptoms Can Worsen As A Result Of Emotional Stress. Techniques For Managing Stress, Such Mindfulness, Meditation, And Relaxation Exercises, May Lessen The Negative Effects Of Stress On Eczema.

5. Weather Report:

• Severe Weather, Especially Dry And Cold Conditions, Can Exacerbate Flare-Ups Of Eczema. It Can Be Beneficial To

Wear Suitable Attire And Protect The Skin In Inclement Weather.

6. Perspiration:

• Persistent Perspiration, Particularly In Regions Where Skin Is Prone To Friction, Can Irritate The Skin And Cause Eczema. Sweating Can Be Remedied By Taking A Shower And Changing Into Fresh, Airy Clothes.

7. Specific Foods:

• Although Less Frequent, Some People's Eczema Symptoms May Be Triggered By Particular Foods. Wheat, Dairy Products, Eggs, And Nuts Are Frequently The Culprits. Keeping A Meal Journal Could Be Useful In Determining Possible Triggers.

8. Changes In Hormones:

• Eczema Symptoms May Be Influenced By Hormonal Changes, Such As Those That Occur During Pregnancy Or Menstruation. During These Hormonal Fluctuations, Women May Detect Changes In Their Skin.

9. Microbiological Infections:

• Fungal, Bacterial, Or Viral Infections Can Make Eczema Worse. Flare-Ups Can Be Avoided By Practicing Proper Cleanliness And Taking Quick Action To Cure Any Skin Infections.

10. Itching:

• Scratching Or Massaging The Afflicted Areas Might Exacerbate The Symptoms Of Eczema And Cause More

Inflammation. To Reduce Skin Damage, It's Critical To Refrain From Excessive Scratching And To Maintain Short Nails.

A Key Component Of Managing Eczema Is Recognizing And Avoiding Its Causes. Working With Medical Specialists To Create A Customized Plan That Targets Their Unique Triggers And Combines Medications And Preventive Measures May Be Beneficial For Those With Eczema.

CHAPTER TWO
Diet's Function In Eczema

There Is No One-Size-Fits-All Solution When It Comes To The Relationship Between Diet And Eczema, Although Some People With The Condition May Find That Specific Food Items Have An Impact On Their Symptoms. It's Crucial To Remember That Different People Have Different Food Triggers, So What Works For One Person Might Not Work For Another. The Following Are Some Factors Pertaining To How Diet Affects Eczema:

1. Allergies To Food:

• Food Allergies May Be A Factor In Flare-Ups For Some Eczema Sufferers. Cow's Milk, Eggs, Peanuts, Tree Nuts,

Soy, Wheat, Fish, And Shellfish Are Among The Common Food Allergies. For Those With Verified Food Allergies, Managing Eczema May Involve Identifying And Removing Particular Allergens From The Diet Under The Supervision Of A Medical Practitioner.

2. Diets Based On Elimination:

• To Find Possible Triggers, Medical Professionals May Advise Exclusion Diets. This Entails Cutting Out Particular Foods From The Diet For A Predetermined Amount Of Time, Then Progressively Adding Them Back In While Keeping An Eye Out For Any Changes In Eczema Symptoms.

3. Anti-Inflammatory Food Plan:

• An Anti-Inflammatory Diet Rich In Foods High In Omega-3 Fatty Acids, Antioxidants, And Anti-Inflammatory Qualities May Be Beneficial For Certain Eczema Sufferers. Fatty Fish, Walnuts, Flaxseeds, Fruits, Vegetables, And Green Tea Are A Few Examples.

4. Probiotics:

• Probiotics Are Good Bacteria That Have The Potential To Improve Gut Health. Probiotics May Be Taken Into Consideration As An Additional Strategy For Treating Eczema Symptoms, As Some Research Points To A Possible Connection Between Gut Health And The Condition.

Nevertheless, Additional Investigation Is Required To Produce Definitive Proof.

5. Drinking Plenty Of Water

• It's Crucial To Drink Enough Water To Be Hydrated In Order To Maintain Good Skin Health Overall. Maintaining Adequate Hydration Helps Avoid Dry Skin, Which Frequently Results In Eczema.

6. Intolerances To Food:

• Although Food Allergies Elicit An Immunological Reaction, Some People May Have Dietary Sensitivity, Which Can Exacerbate Inflammation And Set Off The Symptoms Of Eczema.

Recognizing And Treating Particular Dietary Sensitivity May Be Beneficial.

Before Implementing Major Dietary Changes, People With Eczema Should Speak With Medical Professionals Like Dermatologists Or Allergists. These Experts Can Assist In Determining Whether Particular Food Components Might Be Causing Eczema Symptoms And Can Direct Patients Toward The Right Treatments.

It's Crucial To Understand That Eczema Is A Complicated Disorder Influenced By A Variety Of Factors, Including Genetics, Environment, And Immune System Reactions, Even Though Some People May Benefit From Dietary Changes. An All-

Encompassing Strategy That Includes Good Skincare, Avoiding Triggers, And, If Needed, Dietary Adjustments, May Help Treat Eczema Effectively.

Intolerances And Hypersensitivity

Excessive Sensitivity To Allergens Is A Major Cause Of Eczema And Other Allergic Disorders. In Order To Effectively Manage These Illnesses, It Is Imperative To Distinguish Between Allergies And Sensitivities.

1. Allergens:

• **Definition:** Materials Known As Allergens Have The Ability To Cause An Immunological Reaction In People Who Have Allergies. Even Though These Compounds Are Generally

Harmless, The Immune System Interprets Them As Hazardous And Initiates An Allergic Reaction.

• **Allergic Reaction:** When An Allergic Reaction Occurs, The Body Releases Histamines And Other Substances, Causing Swelling, Redness, Itching, And, In Extreme Situations, Breathing Difficulties Or Anaphylaxis.

• **Common Allergens:** Pollen, Dust Mites, Pet Dander, Nuts, Shellfish, Insect Stings, And Several Drugs Are Examples Of Common Allergens.

2. Sensitivities:

• **Definition:** Sensitivities Are Defined As Negative Responses To Chemicals That Could Not Directly Affect The

Immune System. Sensitivities, In Contrast To Allergies, Do Not Usually Cause An Immunological Response But Can Nevertheless Cause Symptoms That Are Comparable To Those Of Allergies.

- **Reaction:** Sensitivities Can Cause A Range Of Symptoms, Including Headaches, Skin Conditions, Digestive Problems, And General Discomfort. Compared To The Instantaneous And Sometimes Severe Reactions Associated With Allergies, These Reactions Might Be More Subdued.

- **Common Sensitivities:** Common Sensitivities Include Non-Celiac Gluten Sensitivity (Adverse Reactions To Gluten Without Celiac Disease),

Lactose Intolerance (Difficulty Digesting Lactose), And Some Dietary Additives Or Preservatives.

In Relation To Eczema:

• **Food Allergies:** Certain Food Allergies May Aggravate The Symptoms Of Eczema In Certain People. Cow's Milk, Eggs, Peanuts, Tree Nuts, Soy, Wheat, Fish, And Shellfish Are Among The Common Allergies. For Those People, Managing Their Eczema May Involve Recognizing And Avoiding Certain Allergies.

• **Food Sensitivities:** Although They Might Not Directly Trigger An Immunological Reaction, Some People

May Nonetheless Experience Exacerbation Of Eczema Symptoms Due To Food Sensitivities. Common Sensitivities Could Be Allergies To Particular Chemicals Or Components In Processed Foods. Utilizing An Exclusion Diet Or Food Journal May Be Necessary For Identifying And Treating These Sensitivities.

Working Closely With Medical Specialists Like Dermatologists Or Allergists Can Help People With Eczema Discover Particular Allergens Or Sensitivities That May Be Aggravating Their Symptoms. To Identify Triggers, Diagnostic Techniques Such As Skin Testing, Blood Testing, And Elimination Diets

May Be Employed. Once These Triggers Have Been Identified, Avoiding Or Controlling Them Can Be A Crucial Component Of A Successful Eczema Care Strategy.

Creating A Basis For The Healing Of Eczema

Creating A Foundation For Eczema Healing Requires A Multifaceted Strategy That Takes Into Account Potential Triggers, Skincare Regimens, And Lifestyle Choices. The Following Crucial Actions Will Lay The Groundwork For Controlling And Curing Eczema:

1. Speak With Medical Professionals:

• Speak With Dermatologists Or Allergists Who Focus On Skin Disorders As A Starting Point. They Can Assist In Establishing A Customized Treatment Plan, Diagnosing Eczema, And Identifying Particular Triggers.

2. Find And Steer Clear Of Triggers:

• Collaborate With Medical Experts To Determine Any Triggers, Such As Irritants, Allergies, And Sensitivities. This Could Entail Keeping A Food And Symptom Journal, Patch Testing, Or Allergy Testing.

3. Establish A Gentle Skincare Program:

• Use Moisturizers And Moderate Cleansers Without Fragrances To Keep Skin Nourished And Less Irritated. Steer Clear Of Scents, Alcohol-Containing Products, And Harsh Soaps Since These Might Exacerbate Eczema Symptoms.

4. Moisturize Often:

• To Seal In Moisture, Apply Moisturizer To Damp Skin Right Away After Taking A Bath. Select Moisturizers That Are Hypoallergenic And Fragrance-Free To Avoid Drying Out, Which Is A Typical Cause Of Eczema.

5. Make Use Of Non-Irritating Clothes:

• Steer Clear Of Rough Or Scratchy Materials And Opt Instead For Soft, Breathable Materials Like Cotton. To Reduce Irritation, Wash Garments With Gentle, Fragrance-Free Detergents.

6. Steer Clear Of Hot Water:

• Use Lukewarm Water For Your Bath Rather Than Hot, As The Latter Can Exacerbate Dryness And Remove The Skin Of Its Natural Oils. Use Mild Cleansers And Limit Your Bath Duration To Ten To Fifteen Minutes.

7. Control Your Stress:

• Eczema Symptoms Can Be Brought On By Or Made Worse By Stress. To

Assist Manage Stress, Engage In Stress-Relieving Activities Like Yoga, Mindfulness, Deep Breathing Exercises, Or Meditation.

8. Keep Up A Nutritional Diet:

• While Each Person Has Different Dietary Triggers, Eating A Balanced, Nutrient-Rich Diet Can Enhance General Health. In Rare Circumstances, People May Find It Advantageous To Stay Away From Particular Allergies Or Irritants That Have Been Identified After Consulting With Medical Experts.

9. Maintain Hydration:

• To Keep The Body And Skin Hydrated, Drink Enough Water. Staying Properly Hydrated Can Lower

The Chance Of Eczema Flare-Ups And Help Maintain Healthy Skin.

10. Steer Clear Of Scratching:

• Refrain From Scratching, As This Can Aggravate Eczema Symptoms And Cause Skin Damage. Particularly For Kids, Keep Nails Short And Think About Using Anti-Scratch Mittens.

11. Prescription Drugs:

• If Required, Adhere To The Medical Professionals' Recommended Treatment Plan. Topical Steroids, Immunomodulators, And Other Drugs That Reduce Inflammation And Symptoms May Be Included In This.

12. Continual Communication With Medical Professionals:

• Make Appointments For Routine Check-Ups With Medical Professionals To Discuss Any Problems, Track Progress, And Modify Treatment Plans As Necessary.

Establishing A Foundation For The Healing Of Eczema Entails Addressing Lifestyle Issues, Recognizing And Controlling Triggers, And Maintaining Consistency In Skincare Procedures. To Effectively Manage Eczema Over The Long Term And Customize The Strategy To Each Patient's Needs, Close Collaboration With Healthcare Specialists Is Essential.

CHAPTER THREE
How To Develop A Balanced Eczema Diet

A Balanced Eczema Diet Should Emphasize Foods High In Nutrients That Promote Healthy Skin Generally And May Help Lower Inflammation. Remember That Every Person Reacts Differently To Different Foods, So It's Important To Monitor Your Body's Responses And Customize Your Diet In Consultation With Medical Professionals. Here Are Some Broad Pointers For Putting Together A Diet That Is Balanced And Eczema-Friendly:

1. Foods That Reduce Inflammation:

• Add Items With Anti-Inflammatory Qualities To Your Diet. Examples Of Fatty Fish That Are High In Omega-3 Fatty Acids And Can Help Reduce Inflammation Are Trout, Salmon, And Mackerel.

2. Produce And Fruits:

• Eat A Range Of Vibrant Fruits And Vegetables; Their High Antioxidant Content Can Aid In The Fight Against Inflammation. Carrots, Tomatoes, Leafy Greens, And Berries Are Great Options.

3. Complete Grains:

• Choose Whole Grains, Which Provide Fiber And Important Nutrients, Like

Quinoa, Brown Rice, And Oats. Steer Clear Of Refined Carbs And Highly Processed Cereals.

4. Trim Proteins:

• Select Lean Protein Sources From Foods Like Fish, Chicken, Tofu, Lentils, And Nuts. For General Health And Skin Restoration, Protein Is Necessary.

5. Foods High In Probiotics:

• There Is Evidence Linking Skin Issues To Gut Health, And Probiotics May Help Maintain Gut Health. As A Source Of Probiotics, Include Foods Like Yogurt, Kefir, Sauerkraut, Kimchi, And Other Fermented Foods.

6. Good Fats:

• Include Foods Like Avocados, Nuts, Seeds, And Olive Oil That Are Good Sources Of Fat. These Fats Supply Vital Fatty Acids That Promote The Health Of The Skin.

7. Drinking Plenty Of Water

• To Stay Hydrated, Sip Lots Of Water. Drinking Enough Water Will Help Keep Skin Hydrated And Can Stop Dryness, Which Is A Common Cause Of Eczema.

8. Minimize Foods That Could Trigger:

• Be Aware Of Foods That, In Certain Cases, Can Exacerbate Eczema Symptoms. Eggs, Gluten, Dairy, And

Nuts Are Common Causes. Under The Advice Of Medical Experts, Think About Going On An Elimination Diet If You Have Suspicions About Any Particular Foods.

9. Steer Clear Of Highly Processed Foods:

• Reduce The Amount Of Highly Processed Foods You Eat Because They Can Include Preservatives And Additives That Aggravate Inflammation.

10. Meal Journal:

• Maintain A Food Journal To Monitor Dietary Changes And Alterations In Eczema Symptoms. This Can Assist In

Locating Trends And Possible Triggers.

11. Speak With Medical Professionals:

• Speak With Medical Experts, Such As A Certified Dietitian, Allergist, Or Dermatologist, Before Making Any Major Dietary Changes. They Can Offer Tailored Advice Depending On Your Unique Requirements And Possible Triggers.

Keep In Mind That Every Person's Reaction To Food Varies, And There Isn't A Diet That Works For Everyone With Eczema. It's Critical To Concentrate On Eating A Well-Balanced, Nutrient-Rich Diet, Pay

Attention To Your Body's Cues, And Collaborate With Medical Professionals To Customize Your Dietary Regimen To Your Particular Requirements And Dietary Sensitivity.

Recognizing and Steering Clear Of Trigger Foods

Knowing Which Foods To Avoid And Which Ones To Identify As Triggers Is Crucial For Controlling Eczema Symptoms Since For Some People, Certain Foods Can Make Symptoms Worse. The Following Actions Can Be Taken To Recognize And Get Rid Of Possible Trigger Foods:

1. Maintain A Food Journal:

• To Begin, Keep A Thorough Food Journal For A Few Weeks. Keep Track Of Everything You Consume, Including Condiments And Snacks. Take Note Of The Serving Sizes And Timing As Well.

2. Monitor Symptoms:

• Note The Intensity Of Your Eczema Symptoms In Addition To Your Food Journal. Keep An Eye Out For Any Modifications Or Escalation Of Skin Complaints.

3. Seek Out Trends:

• Examine Your Food Journal And Eczema Symptom Logs For Any Possible Trends Or Connections. Seek Out Situations In Which Alterations In

Eczema Symptoms Correspond With The Ingestion Of Particular Foods.

4. Typical Foods That Trigger:

• Although Trigger Foods Might Differ From Person To Person, Dairy Products, Eggs, Almonds, Seeds, Soy, Wheat, Fish, And Shellfish Are Frequently The Cause For Certain Persons. Preservatives And Food Additives May Further Exacerbate The Symptoms Of Eczema.

5. Examine Sensitivities And Allergies:

• To Investigate The Possibilities Of Food Allergies Or Sensitivities, Speak With Medical Specialists Like Dermatologists Or Allergists. Testing

For Allergies, Such As Blood Or Skin Tests, Can Be Used To Pinpoint Certain Triggers.

6. Diet of Elimination:

• Take Into Consideration Working With Medical Specialists To Develop An Elimination Diet. This Is Taking Foods That May Be Triggers Out Of Your Diet For A Short While, Then Returning Them One At A Time While Keeping An Eye Out For Any Changes In Your Symptoms.

7. Keep An Eye Out For Non-Food Triggers:

• In Addition To Diet, Be Mindful Of Potential Triggers From The Surroundings (Dust Mites, Pollen,

Etc.), Skincare Products, Stress, And Weather.

8. Speak With A Qualified Nutritionist:

• A Qualified Dietician Can Offer Professional Advice On Recognizing And Avoiding Trigger Foods. They Can Assist You In Putting Together A Nutritious, Well-Balanced Diet That Stays Away From Possible Triggers.

9. Examine Food Labels:

• Pay Close Attention To Food Labels To Find Any Allergens Or Substances That Can Aggravate Eczema Symptoms. Common Allergies May Have Hidden Sources In Some Packaged Goods.

10. Reintroduction Gradually:

• Reintroduce Foods One At A Time And Gradually If You Have Eliminated Them. By Using This Method, You'll Be Able to Identify Particular Triggers and Improve Your Diet Management.

11. Be Persistent and Patient:

• It May Take Some Time To Identify Trigger Foods, And Persistence And Patience May Be Needed. Dietary Changes Might Not Show Results Right Away, So Constant Observation And Tweaking Are Crucial.

Keep In Mind That Every Person's Body Responds Differently, And That Different People Can Have Different Trigger Foods. To Make Sure You Are

Still Fulfilling Your Nutritional Demands, It Is Imperative To Undertake Dietary Adjustments Under The Supervision Of Medical Professionals. Additionally, Even Though Some Foods Must Be Restricted Or Avoided, Eating A Balanced, Nutrient-Rich Diet Is Crucial For Good Health Overall.

CHAPTER THREE
Particular Attention to Children Affected By Eczema

Children's Eczema Management Calls For Particular Attention Because Of Their Special Needs And Difficulties. Here Are Some Particular Things Parents And Other Caregivers Should Keep In Mind When Managing A Child's Eczema:

1. Mild Skincare:

• For Children, Use Gentle, Fragrance-Free, And Hypoallergenic Skincare Products. Steer Clear Of Abrasive Detergents And Soaps That Might Irritate Skin. After Giving Them A Quick Wash In Warm Water, Moisturize Them Right Away.

2. Options for Clothes:

• Clothe Kids In Cotton Or Other Gentle, Breathable Materials. Steer Clear Of Wool And Synthetic Materials That Can Irritate Your Skin. Use Mild Detergents Without Fragrances While Washing Their Clothing.

3. Cut Nails:

• Cut Your Child's Nails Short To Reduce The Possibility Of Them Scratching And Hurting Their Skin. To Stop Children From Scratching At Night, Especially The Smaller Ones, You Might Also Think About Wearing Soft Mittens.

4. Suitable Moisturizing Routine for Children:

• Create A Consistent Moisturizing Regimen. Make It Enjoyable And Fulfilling For The Kids To Make It Kid-Friendly. Make It A Fun Activity To Choose Their Moisturizer Together.

5. Keep Common Allergens Away:

• Recognize And Steer Clear Of Common Food Allergies That Could Aggravate Your Child's Eczema Symptoms. Cow's Milk, Eggs, Peanuts, Tree Nuts, Soy, Wheat, Fish, And Shellfish Are Among The Common Allergies.

6. Wearing Protective Clothes:

• Wear Clothes On Your Child To Protect Them From Chilly Temperatures And Strong Winds During The Winter. As The Inner Layer, Choose Breathable Materials To Prevent Perspiration, Which Can Aggravate Eczema.

7. Teach Teachers And Caregivers:

• Share with Caregivers, Educators, and Other Adults Who Interact With Your Child Information Regarding Their Skincare Regimen, Particular Considerations, And Triggers For Eczema. This Guarantees Uniformity In The Treatment Of Eczema In Various Settings.

8. Remain Alert For Environmental Stressors:

• Recognize Environmental Triggers, Including Pollen, Pet Dander, And Dust Mites. Make Sure Your Child's Room Is Tidy And Take Precautions Like Using Pillowcases And Mattresses That Are Allergen-Proof.

9. Speak With A Pediatric Dermatologist:

• See A Pediatric Dermatologist If Your Child Has Severe Or Chronic Eczema. They Can Offer Customized Therapy Plans And Expert Advice For Kids.

10. Control Your Stress:

• Stress Can Aggravate The Symptoms Of Eczema In Children. Promote

Stress-Relieving Pursuits Including Leisure, Recreation, And Getting Enough Sleep.

11. Collaborate With The School:

• If Your Child Attends School, Work With The Instructors And Other Staff Members To Make Sure They Are Informed About Your Child's Illness. Talk About Any Necessary Modifications, Such Using Fragrance-Free Products Or Having The Go-Ahead To Use Moisturizer During The Day.

12. Get Emotional Assistance:

• Coping With Long-Term Illnesses Can Be Emotionally Taxing For Both Caregivers And Kids. Seek Emotional

Assistance To Manage The Emotional Components Of Managing Eczema, Such As Through Therapy Or Support Groups.

Keep In Mind That Each Child Is Different, So What Suits One Might Not Suit Another. Creating A Customized And Successful Management Strategy For Your Child's Eczema Requires Close Collaboration With Medical Specialists, Such As Dermatologists And Pediatricians.

Lifestyle Elements and the Management of Eczema

Lifestyle Choices Can Directly Affect The Frequency And Intensity Of Flare-Ups, Which Is Important For Controlling Eczema. The Following Important Lifestyle Factors Can Help With Eczema Management:

1. Skincare Regimen:

• Create A Moderate And Regular Skincare Regimen. To Keep The Skin Hydrated Use Gentle Cleansers And Moisturizers Without Fragrance. Steer Clear Of Abrasive Soaps And Detergents That May Deplete The Skin's Natural Oils.

2. Wetness:

• Consistent Miniaturization Is Essential For Managing Eczema. To Seal In Moisture, Apply A Moisturizer Right Away After Taking A Bath. Select Items That Are Fragrance-Free And Hypoallergenic.

3. Steer Clear Of Triggers:

• Recognize And Stay Away From Triggers That Might Make Eczema Symptoms Worse. Allergens, Irritants, And Sensitivities Fall Under This Category. Collaborate With Medical Experts To Identify Certain Triggers.

4. Nutritional Points to Remember:

• Monitor Your Diet And Take Into Account Any Dietary Triggers. While

Some Eczema Sufferers May Benefit From An Anti-Inflammatory Diet, Others May Need To Stay Away From Particular Allergies Or Sensitivities.

5. Drinking Plenty of Water

• Make Sure You're Getting Enough Water To Stay Hydrated. Staying Well Hydrated Will Help Avoid Dryness, Which Is A Common Cause Of Eczema, And Preserve The General Health Of The Skin.

6. Options for Clothes:

• Wear Loose, Airy Clothing, Such As Cotton, And Stay Away From Anything Too Tight Or Itchy. To Lessen The Chance Of Irritation, Wash Items In Gentle, Fragrance-Free Detergents.

7. Humidity and Temperature:

• Control Humidity And Temperature To Keep A Cozy Atmosphere Inside. Severe Weather Conditions Might Exacerbate Eczema Flare-Ups.

8. Handling Stress:

• Engage In Stress-Relieving Activities Like Yoga, Mindfulness, Deep Breathing, Or Meditation. Since Stress Can Worsen The Symptoms Of Eczema, Stress Management Is Essential To General Wellbeing.

9. Frequent Workout:

• To Improve General Health, Engage In Moderate Activity On A Regular Basis. Avoid Engaging In Activities That Could Lead To Excessive

Perspiration, And Take A Quick Shower Afterward To Prevent Irritation.

10. Sufficient Sleep:

• Make Sure You Receive Plenty Good Sleep. Sleep Deprivation Can Exacerbate Stress And Have An Adverse Effect On The Immune System, Which May Affect The Symptoms Of Eczema.

11. Environmental Allergens:

• Recognize Allergens In The Surroundings, Such As Dust Mites, Pollen, And Pet Dander. Reduce Exposure By Employing Tools Like Air Purifiers And Bedding That Is Allergy-Proof.

12. Speak With Medical Professionals:

• Consult Dermatologists, Allergists, Or Other Medical Specialists On A Regular Basis To Evaluate Your Eczema And Modify Your Treatment Strategy As Necessary.

13. Steer Clear Of Smoke And Secondhand Smoke:

• Secondhand Smoke Exposure And Smoking Can Exacerbate Eczema Symptoms. If You Smoke, Think About Giving It Up And Stay Away From Tobacco Smoke.

14. Teach Your Friends And Family:

• Make Sure Your Friends And Family Are Informed Of Your Eczema

Treatment Plan, As Well As Any Special Requirements Or Accommodations You Might Need.

An All-Encompassing Strategy That Takes Into Account These Lifestyle Factors Can Help With Eczema Management. Working Together With Healthcare Providers Is Crucial To Creating A Customized Strategy That Takes Into Account Your Particular Needs And Triggers. Maintaining Regular Contact With Your Healthcare Team Guarantees Continued Support And Allows For Any Necessary Modifications To Your Management Plan.

CHAPTER FOUR
Supplements To Help With Eczema

Although A Well-Balanced Diet Is The Best Way To Obtain Vital Nutrients, Some Eczema Sufferers Might Think About Taking Supplements To Help Their Skin. Since Everyone's Demands Are Different, It Is Imperative That You Speak With Medical Professionals Before Incorporating Any Supplements Into Your Regimen. The Following Supplements Have Been Recommended To Help With Eczema:

1. The Fatty Acids Omega-3:

• Fish Oil Supplements, Which Are High In Omega-3 Fatty Acids, May Help Eczema Because Of Their Potential Anti-Inflammatory Effects. To Find Out

The Right Dosage, Speak With A Medical Practitioner.

2. Probiotics:

• Supplements Containing Probiotics Include Good Bacteria That Promote Intestinal Health. Certain Skin Problems, Like Eczema, May Be Related To Gut Health, According To Certain Data. Probiotics Could Be Viewed As An Additional Strategy For Managing Eczema.

3. Vitamin D:

• Vitamin D Is Important For Immune System Performance, And There May Be A Link Between Eczema And Vitamin D Insufficiency, According To Certain Research. Still, Further

Investigation Is Required To Prove A Certain Connection. In The Event Of A Deficiency, A Medical Practitioner Might Suggest Supplements.

4. Zinc:

• Zinc Is A Necessary Mineral That Affects Wound Healing And Skin Health. Lower Zinc Levels May Be Present In Some Eczema Sufferers. But Taking Too Much Zinc Might Have Negative Effects, Therefore Professional Advice Should Be Sought Before Beginning Any Supplementation.

5. Vitamin E:

• An Antioxidant Called Vitamin E May Help Maintain The General Health Of

The Skin. Although There Isn't Much Data On How Specifically It Affects Eczema, It Can Be Helpful To Include Foods High In Vitamin E In Your Diet Or Think About Taking Supplements Under Medical Supervision.

6. Quercetin:

• A Flavonoid Having Anti-Inflammatory And Antioxidant Qualities Is Quercetin. According To Certain Research, It Might Aid In Immune Response Modulation, Which Might Be Advantageous For Eczema Sufferers. In Addition To Supplements, Quercetin Can Be Found In Foods Like Apples, Onions, And Berries.

7. Borage Oil:

• Gamma-Linolenic Acid (GLA), An Omega-6 Fatty Acid, Is Present In Boreage Oil. GLA Might Help Some People With Eczema Since It Has Anti-Inflammatory Qualities. Like Other Supplements, Though, It Should Only Be Taken Under Medical Supervision.

It's Crucial To Remember That Supplements Shouldn't Take The Place Of A Balanced Diet; Instead, Their Use Should Be Determined By The Demands And Deficiencies Of Each Individual. The Right Dosage For A Given Vitamin Or Mineral Should Be Determined In Consultation With Healthcare Professionals As

Overdosing On Them Might Have Negative Effects.

Furthermore, There Is Not Always Strong Evidence To Support The Effectiveness Of Specific Supplements, Even Though Some People May Find Them To Be Helpful In Relieving Eczema Symptoms. Supplementation Should Always Be Used In Conjunction With A Comprehensive Eczema Management Plan That Takes Good Skincare, Lifestyle Choices, And Expert Advice Into Account.

Recipes for Eczema Healing

While There Isn't A Specific Set Of Recipes Guaranteed To Heal Eczema, Incorporating Nutrient-Dense And Anti-Inflammatory Foods Into Your Diet May Help Support Overall Skin Health. Here Are A Few Recipes That Emphasize Ingredients Believed To Be Beneficial For Individuals With Eczema:

1. Recipe for Omega-3 Rich Salmon with Quinoa and Vegetables: Ingredients:

- Salmon Fillets
- Quinoa
- Broccoli
- Cherry Tomatoes

- Olive Oil
- Lemon Juice
- Garlic
- Salt And Pepper

Instructions: Bake or Grill Salmon Fillets Seasoned With Olive Oil, Lemon Juice, Garlic, Salt, and Pepper.

- Cook Quinoa As Directed On The Package.

- Steam The Broccoli Until It Is Soft.

- Mix Quinoa With Steamed Broccoli And Cherry Tomatoes.

- Place The Salmon On Top Of The Quinoa And Vegetable Mixture.

2. Anti-Inflammatory Smoothie:

Ingredients:

- 1 Cup Of Berries (Blueberries, Strawberries, Or Raspberries)
- 1 Banana
- 1 Tablespoon Of Chia Seeds
- 1 Tablespoon Of Flaxseed Meal
- 1 Cup of Spinach Or Kale
- 1 Cup Of Unsweetened Almond Milk Or Coconut Water

Instructions: Combine All Ingredients And Blend Until A Smooth Consistency Is Achieved.

Adjust the Consistency by Adding Additional Liquid If Necessary.

3. Avocado and Spinach Salad: Ingredients:

Spinach Leaves

Cherry Tomatoes

Cucumber

Avocado

Grilled Chicken Breast (Optional) Olive Oil and Balsamic Vinegar Dressing

Instructions: Combine Spinach Leaves With Sliced Cherry Tomatoes, Cucumber, And Avocado.

• Include Grilled Chicken If Preferred.

• Drizzle With Olive Oil And Balsamic Vinegar Dressing.

4. Turmeric Ginger Carrot Soup:

Ingredients:

- Chopped Carrots
- Chopped Onion
- Minced Garlic
- Grated Fresh Ginger
- Ground Turmeric
- Vegetable Or Chicken Broth - Coconut Milk
- Olive Oil
- Salt and Pepper

• Sauté Onions, Garlic, and Ginger in Olive Oil Until They Are Softened.

• Add Diced Carrots And Sauté Further.

• Add Ground Turmeric And Mix Well.

• Add The Broth And Cook Until The Carrots Are Soft.

• Blend The Soup Until It Reaches A Smooth Consistency, Then Incorporate The Coconut Milk.

Season with Salt and Pepper According To Your Preference.

5. Quinoa And Kale Stuffed Bell Peppers:

Ingredients:

Bell Peppers, Halved And Deseeded

Quinoa Chopped Kale Drained And Rinsed Black Beans

• Diced Tomato

• Sliced Avocado

- Cumin, Paprika, And Garlic Powder

- Olive Oil

- Lime Juice

  - Cook Quinoa as Per the Instructions on the Package.
  - Sauté Kale in Olive Oil Until It Wilts.
  - Combine Cooked Quinoa, Black Beans, Sautéed Kale, Diced Tomato, And Spices In A Bowl.
  - Fill The Bell Peppers With The Quinoa Mixture.
  - Bake Until the Peppers Are Soft.
  - Top With Sliced Avocado And A Drizzle Of Lime Juice.

Remember That Individual Responses To Specific Foods Can Vary, And It's

Essential To Consult With Healthcare Professionals For Personalized Dietary Advice. These Recipes Emphasize Nutrient-Dense And Anti-Inflammatory Ingredients That May Support Overall Skin Health, But They Are Not A Substitute For Professional Medical Advice And Treatment.

Snacks and Desserts

Selecting Ingredients For Desserts And Snacks That Are Less Likely To Cause Eczema Symptoms Is Important For Those Who Have The Condition. These Dessert And Snack Alternatives Are Suitable For Those With Eczema:

1. Berry Parfait: Mixed Berries (Strawberries, Raspberries, And Blueberries)

• Coconut Yogurt Or Dairy-Free Yogurt

- Granola (If Necessary, Gluten-Free)
- Honey, If Desired

• To Prepare, Top A Glass With Granola, Dairy-Free Yogurt, And Mixed Berries.

• Repeat With The Layers.

• If Desired, Drizzle With Honey.

2. Baked Apple Chips:

Ingredients:

• Thinly Cut Apples

- Ground Cinnamon

- Optional Coconut Oil

Directions:

1. Set Oven Temperature To 200°F, Or 93°C.
2. Toss Apple Slices With A Tiny Bit Of Melted Coconut Oil And A Dash Of Cinnamon, If Preferred.
3. Place Slices In A Single Layer On A Baking Sheet.
4. Bake the Chips for 2 To 3 Hours, Or Until They Are Crisp.

3. Banana-Oat Cookies:

- **Ingredients:** Mashed Ripe Bananas Rolled Oats Cinnamon Vanilla Extract Optional Nuts Or Seeds

- **Directions:**

  - Set Oven Temperature To 350°F (175°C).

  - Combine Mashed Bananas, Rolled Oats, Vanilla Essence, A Pinch Of Cinnamon, And Any Nuts Or Seeds You Choose In A Bowl.

  - Spoon Mixture Onto A Baking Sheet In Spoonfuls.

  - Bake For 12 To 15 Minutes, Or Until Golden Brown Around The Edges.

4. Avocado Chocolate Mousse:

- **Ingredients:**

- Pitted And Peeling Ripe Avocados

• Powdered Cocoa Without Sugar

• Honey Or Maple Syrup

• Vanilla Extract

• To Make The Recipe, Blend Together Avocados, Cocoa Powder, Vanilla Essence, And Maple Syrup Or Honey Until Smooth.

• Taste And Adjust Sweetness.

• Let Cool For A Minimum Of Half An Hour Prior To Serving.

5. Trail Mix:

• Components:

- Nuts (Almonds, Cashews, Or Walnuts)
- Seeds (Sunflower, Pumpkin)

- Dried Fruit (Apricots, Cranberries)
- Dark Chocolate Chips

Directions: In A Bowl, Combine Dark Chocolate Chips, Almonds, Seeds, And Dried Fruit.

- Transfer into Convenient Little Snack-Sized Bags.

6. Almond Flour And Shredded Coconut Are The Ingredients For Coconut Bliss Balls.

- Pitted Medjool Dates
- Vanilla Essence
- Almond Butter

- **Directions:** Process Almond Butter, Shredded Coconut, Pitted Dates,

Almond Flour, Vanilla Essence, and Almond Butter In A Food Processor until A Dough Forms.

• Form The Mixture Into Tiny Balls And Store Them In The Fridge.

7. Rice Cake with Banana and Almond Butter: Rice Cakes As An Ingredient

- Almond Butter
- A Sliced Banana

• **Directions:** Spread Rice Cake With Almond Butter.

• Add Slices Of Banana On Top.

Ingredients In These Snacks And Desserts Are Less Likely To Aggravate Eczema Symptoms. Individual

Sensitivities Can Differ, Though, So It's Important To Be Aware Of How Your Body Responds And Seek The Assistance Of Medical Professionals For Specific Guidance.

Conclusion

In Summary, Treating Eczema Requires A Multimodal Strategy That Takes Into Account Environmental Influences, Food Choices, Skincare Practices, And Lifestyle Considerations. Effective Eczema Management Can Be Achieved By Implementing Techniques To Detect And Prevent Triggers, Maintain Regular Skincare, Adopt A Balanced Diet, Manage Stress, And Seek Professional Help. However, There Is No One-Size-Fits-All Answer.

• To Keep The Skin Hydrated And Less Irritated, Gentle Cleaning And Frequent Moisturizing Should Be The Main Goals Of Skincare Regimens.

Minimizing Flare-Ups Can Be Achieved By Identifying And Avoiding Triggers, Such As Allergens And Irritants, Using Techniques Like Allergy Testing And Elimination Diets. In Addition, Sustaining An Anti-Inflammatory Diet That Is Well-Balanced, Drinking Plenty Of Water, Controlling Stress, And Getting Enough Sleep Are Critical For Promoting General Skin Health.

• It's Important To Speak With Medical Specialists Before Making Any Dietary Changes Or Supplement Decisions To Make Sure Specific Demands Are Satisfied And Hazards Are Kept To A Minimum. Furthermore, Keeping Lines Of Communication Open With Allergists, Dermatologists, And Other

Medical Professionals Enables Continuous Assessment And Necessary Modifications To The Treatment Plan.

A Comprehensive And Individualized Approach To Managing Eczema Can Help People Reduce Symptoms, Improve The Health Of Their Skin, And Feel Better Overall. Keep In Mind That Treating Eczema Is A Journey, And That Figuring Out The Best Mix Of Tactics May Call For Perseverance, Patience, And Support From Family, Friends, And Medical Experts.

THE END